Adrenal Fatigue

Complete Guide of How to Overcoming Adrenal Fatigue Syndrome Naturally, Reduce Stress and Boost Your Energy Levels

Jack Oliver

2016 Edition

I am grateful to my family for their help and support that was provided to me during the making of this little writing.

My father, wife and children dedicated.

P.S. You need to be patient, to go the way of healing with maximum efficiency.

Copyright © 2016 by Kate Murray. All Rights Reserved.
No part of this book may be reproduced, stored in retrieval systems, or transmitted by any means, electronic, mechanical, photocopying, recorded or otherwise without written permission from the author.

Printed Edition
ISBN-13: 978-1539006022
ISBN-10: 1539006026

CONTENT

Overview

What is Adrenal Fatigue?
1. How the depletion of adrenal looks?
2. What happens when our adrenal glands tired?

Little-Known Signs of Adrenal Fatigue

How Do You Know That You Have Adrenal Fatigue?
1. Increased Fatigue
2. Drowsiness and Fatigue - Symptoms of Neurasthenia
3. Chronic Fatigue - a Consequence of Tissue Hypoxia
4. Muscle Fatigue
5. Mental Fatigue. Asthenia
6. Fatigue Eye. Asthenia
7. Spring Fatigue
8. During Pregnancy
9. The Child Has
10. Diagnostics

Three Stages of Adrenal Fatigue
- Stress
- Fatigue
- Exhaustion

Recovery Treatment

Natural Ways to Treat Adrenal Fatigue
- Vitamins
- Water treatment procedures
- Honey Treatment

Choose Proper Diet
- The right time for adrenal health food
- Meals and drinks for the health of the adrenal glands
- Other nutrients needed for the health of the adrenal glands

Epilogue

Author Page
Additional Content

OVERVIEW

Increased fatigue

It's a feeling of complete exhaustion of energy, in which very sleepy or just lie down. This is a natural reaction of the body with a very heavy physical labor in poor holiday or emotionally straining. But sometimes the fatigue talking about diseases of the body or the mind. It is this symptom, often, there is only one. In this case, even a good long rest, and does not help to reduce fatigue. If the fatigue caused by the disease, it can last as long as you want without improvement, regardless of the rest. And sometimes long periods of fatigue may be interleaved sharp rise in activity.

Fatigue - this is normal for teenagers in puberty. However, an important role in this case is the psychological environment in which the child lives. Sometimes, during a depression, triggered by problems with their studies or their parents, the child may sleep for a long time - it is a defense mechanism used by the body.

Sometimes the fatigue is associated with metabolic disorders. If the nutrients are processed body too quickly and does not have time to use them as an energy source or recycled if they are too long. Such a violation may be due to the change in hormone levels, and with malnutrition.

WHAT IS ADRENAL FATIGUE?

You constantly feel tired, without apparent reason? You feel depressed in stressful situations and can't find the strength and energy, which have recently been your business card? You are struggling to bring himself to get out of bed in the morning without feeling rested, even after a long sleep? If you notice any of these symptoms are, most likely you are suffering from adrenal exhaustion.

Depletion of the adrenal glands is a condition provoked adrenal stress, which occurs if the hypothalamus, pituitary and adrenal glands (together - the HPA axis) operate below their optimal functional parameters. Although you may not even have heard of the adrenal glands, they perform several vital functions for the optimal operation of our body. The most important function of the adrenal gland is the body's response to stress in a stressful situation, the adrenal glands secrete into the blood hormones such as cortisol, DHEA and adrenaline, which support the important parameters such as heart rate, immune system, energy storage, and many more.

When stimulated adrenal excessively over a long period, they get tired. Typical cause's adrenal exhaustion include working under stressful conditions, problems in his personal life and chronic diseases. In the end, the adrenal glands are depleted to such an extent that it is not able to respond adequately when we need them. Currently, many suffering from adrenal exhaustion, complain of a feeling of constant fatigue, lack of enthusiasm and moderate depression. For many hours of sleep do not help - they wake up the same tired, however we went to bed. They are normally often consume large amounts of caffeinated beverages, soft drinks or other stimulants to somehow work day.

Adrenal dysfunction is not recognized by modern medicine until it becomes life-threatening when the adrenal glands practically cease to function altogether and becomes an autoimmune disease called Addison's disease. But, the fact that many doctors (at least some of them) are not able to understand, it is a fact that millions of us suffer from a reduced adrenal performance. Simply put, the adrenal glands and some internal organs are still functioning, but a lot less than the proper level. That's no reason to run a hospital emergency room, but it is certainly a big problem for those who are suffering from low adrenal function.

So how can we cure adrenal exhaustion? It's not as simple as take a pill, but it is certainly possible. By making simple changes in your lifestyle that will give the adrenal glands time required for recovery, you could return to its former energy and vitality. First, let's understand what is adrenal exhaustion and how we can recognize it.

How the depletion of adrenal looks?

Adrenal depletion leads to a wide range of symptoms, therefore it is often called a syndrome. However, in simple terms adrenal fatigue can be defined as:

The group of symptoms that occur when the adrenal glands and the HPA-axis function below the optimal level.

Each of these symptoms may be caused by a deficiency of one or several hormones produced by the adrenal glands. The opinions of experts about the term defining this condition are still going. Some of them believe that the term "adrenal exhaustion" is not the most suitable for this condition. Some health experts refer to it as a dysfunction of the HPA axis to stress or adrenal glands. Whatever term is used, be sure that we are talking about the same state. The term adrenal exhaustion is one of the most commonly used.

The most common symptom of adrenal exhaustion is fatigue, but it differs from the usual fatigue that we all experience from time to time. Fatigue caused by the depletion of the adrenal glands, it causes sufferers to have trouble every morning, getting out of bed, even after a long sleep. There is one exception; many patients with adrenal exhaustion feel increased energy levels late in the evening, a phenomenon that is associated with the violation of the cycle of cortisol secretion.

They also complained of a general lack of energy, difficulty to "lift themselves" for any major events, and inability to cope with stressful situations. When the adrenals become fatigued, they lose their ability to produce stress hormones - those that our body uses to reflex response to stress, the type of "fight or flight". This means that many patients with adrenal exhaustion of complaining about the strange feeling of "indifference" in the moments when they should be happy. In addition, it is very difficult to maintain the necessary concentration and energy level, when there are stressful situations, which require hard work.

Other adrenal exhaustion symptoms include cravings for salty foods, low blood sugar, complaints of the respiratory system, allergies, low sex drive, and weight gain. All of this may be due to reduced levels of a hormone produced by the adrenal glands.

What happens when our adrenal glands tired?

You might recognize the symptoms of adrenal exhaustion, but what actually happens to our bodies when we are experiencing the symptoms? Historically, that the depletion of the adrenal glands diagnose only its symptoms. Nowadays, thanks to modern laboratory tests, and a better understanding of human anatomy, we can determine exactly what happens when the patient is suffering from adrenal insufficiency. This helps medical professionals diagnose and treat adrenal fatigue is much more effective.

Understanding the HPA axis is crucial for the understanding of adrenal exhaustion. The adrenal glands are, in this context, part of the network of the three bodies, collectively known as the HPA axis, which determines the level of hormones in our bodies. These three bodies are the hypothalamus, pituitary and adrenal glands.

In a stressful situation, the hypothalamus sends a message to the pituitary gland, which in turn sends a message to the adrenal glands. These causes the adrenal glands secrete stress hormones such as cortisol and adrenaline, which increases blood sugar levels, increase heart rate and blood pressure. Within seconds, your body is ready for a factor, which causes us stress. This is known as an instinctive response to the "fight or flight".

This stress response has evolved to protect us from predators and other immediate threats. However, it is not adapted to respond to the constant stress the low level of modern life that cause a much longer-term increase in the level of stress hormones.

The adrenal glands can quickly recover from a short burst of stress hormone production. But if the stress continues for a long period of time, they are rapidly depleted, with no remaining primary material (cholesterol), which they need for the development of stress hormones. There are compensation mechanisms that allow you to keep for some time the desired level of hormones, but in the end, the level of adrenaline and cortisol yet fall.

It may be noted that the depletion of adrenal multilevel process. First, there is increase in the level of stress hormones to unacceptable levels. After a while, your body responds by lowering production levels of sex hormones to maintain elevated levels of stress hormones. And then, in the next stage, the level of stress hormones starts to fall, because our adrenal glands become unable to handle the load.

Reduced levels of cortisol and adrenaline, coupled with impaired cortisol day cycle, are the cause of many symptoms of adrenal exhaustion. Fatigue, inability to concentrate, sleep disorders cycles and many other symptoms can easily be associated with reduced levels of stress hormones. Other symptoms, such as low sex drive, connected with the violation of the hormonal cascade in the pituitary-adrenal axis. And, seemingly unrelated symptoms such as frequent urination, and a craving for salty foods may be associated with reduced levels of aldosterone, another hormone produced by the adrenal glands.

Perception and linking these disparate symptoms requires experience and knowledge of how our endocrine system works. Fortunately, modern laboratory tests (such as saliva test for cortisol levels) offers us a very useful diagnostic tool. However, the correct interpretation of the test results is very important, as the range of reference values is very wide. Hospital staff, to which you refer, must be very experienced in the diagnosis of adrenal exhaustion.

LITTLE-KNOWN SIGNS OF ADRENAL FATIGUE

1. Dependence on sunglasses.

Sunglasses in the summer - this is not essential and necessary element of many people.

But few know that the eyes hypersensitive to bright sunlight is a sign of problems with the adrenal glands.

Their normal work does not allow a chronic imbalance of sodium - potassium, which prevents pupils from bright sunlight narrowing them properly.

The good news is that being in the midday sun without sunglasses is one of the ways to strengthen the adrenal glands.

When you change the diet, avoid the use of sugar and reduce the carbohydrates from your diet your eyes become less sensitive to sunlight.

But, we should not give up the sunglasses while you are driving a car for safety reasons, to reduce glare.

2. Sunken cheeks.

If you find that your cheeks disappear, become hollow, do not even think about collagen injections or other injections of beauty.

This is a sign of adrenal insufficiency.

You no longer help the rejection of sugar, caffeine and a good sleep.

3. The condition of the skin on the fingers.

Examine the skin on the fingertips from the palm rest.

If you see a good, plump finger-tips, it is a good sign of the presence of adrenal fatigue.

The presence of vertical lines on the fingertips indicates adrenal stress.

4. Pale lips.

If you think that if the lips are pale, it is the age.

You are wrong.

Pale lips that do not have color - it is a sign of weak adrenal glands!

Experts say that if women are excluded from the food grains (gluten free food), refined sugar and caffeine; then again see his pink lips.

5. Balding shin.

Men often have the hair on his arms and legs. If there appears a receding hairline or they become scarcer, it may be a sign of adrenal fatigue.

Boys entering puberty, begin to shave.

If they have a little hair on the feet (or hands), then they reduced adrenal function.

6. Muscle weakness or pain in the knees.

Muscle weakness is often a sign of adrenal insufficiency.

Knee pain without accompanying structural defect may indicate a weakness of the muscles that support the knees.

In the case of back pain, chronic adrenal stress leads to weakness in the muscles that support the pelvis.

In other words, back pain often have nothing to do with the lower part of the back, and is due to muscle imbalance in the pelvis.

HOW DO YOU KNOW THAT YOU HAVE ADRENAL FATIGUE?

Often, fatigue is one of the symptoms of chronic fatigue syndrome. In rare cases, fatigue is a particular individual characteristic of the nervous system. In this case, it is evident from an early age. These babies are very calm, never playing in a noisy and outdoor games for a long time, they are passive and often in a bad mood.

Often, fatigue is caused by certain factors, such as stress, illness, emotional tension, change in activity. If fatigue is associated with CFS, it is necessarily combined with the inability to concentrate, frequent headaches, lethargy, irritability, sleep disorders in which a person can't sleep at night, and all day walking sleepy.

Against the background of such a depressed state at the deteriorating human health - body weight changes, he may start drinking for relaxation, pain in the back and joints, indifference to everything, often aggravated skin diseases, allergies.

Other symptoms of chronic fatigue syndrome:

- Deterioration of concentration,
- Headache,
- Sore throat,
- Enlarged and painful lymph nodes,
- Lethargy, not passing up to six months,
- The lack of freshness and activity after sleep
- Tired after a very small voltage.

Unfortunately, no analysis will not find a violation of health in such a patient. Man has taken on a powerful load of problems, which can't cope, trying to be the best anywhere and get a result of chronic fatigue syndrome. The doctor usually makes the diagnosis "neuro disorder." Moreover, treatment is usually not very helpful. The treatment in this case must be complex.

Increased Fatigue

It's a feeling of complete exhaustion of energy, in which very sleepy or just lie down. This is a natural reaction of the body with a very heavy physical labor in poor holiday or emotionally straining. But sometimes the fatigue talking about diseases of the body or the mind.

It is this symptom, often, there is only one? In this case, even a good long rest, and does not help to reduce fatigue. If the fatigue caused by the disease, it can last as long as you want without improvement, regardless of the rest. And sometimes long periods of fatigue may be interleaved sharp rise in activity.

Fatigue - this is normal for teenagers in puberty. However, an important role in this case is the psychological environment in which the child lives. Sometimes, during a depression, triggered by problems with their studies or their parents, the child may sleep for a long time - it is a defense mechanism used by the body.

Sometimes the fatigue is associated with metabolic disorders. If the nutrients are processed body too quickly and does not have time to use them as an energy source or recycled if they are too long. Such a violation may be due to the change in hormone levels, and with malnutrition.

Drowsiness and Fatigue - Symptoms of Neurasthenia

The combination of these two symptoms often indicate the presence of so-called neurotic symptom or fatigue. This is a very common condition that occurs in one third of patients with neuroses. These patients are very sensitive to harsh noise, bright light, they often have a headache, they sickened, they feel tired even after resting.

The patient does not feel self-confidence, he is anxious and can not relax. He was hard to concentrate and therefore he becomes distracted, operation of such a patient is greatly reduced. In addition, the patient may be disturbed function of digestion. These symptoms are typical for hyposthenia form of neurasthenia.

Chronic Fatigue - a Consequence of Tissue Hypoxia

Thirty years ago, no one knew about chronic fatigue or tiredness. The occurrence of this phenomenon is explained by the frantic strain on the body, including psychological. The higher the load, the greater the need for oxygen. But where to get more? Therefore, every modern man suffers from a lack of oxygen in the tissues. This status entails a violation of metabolism: increased use of glycogen in the body accumulates lactic acid, amino acids and hormones. That is, the metabolic processes are slowed down, and the exchange of products are not derived from the tissue.

In this state the immune system can't protect the body against viruses, bacteria and fungi. Under normal conditions, all of these pathogenic agents are easily destroyed by immune cells. From this situation, there are only two options: to supply sufficient oxygen organism or reduce the intensity of stress.

Muscle Fatigue

Fatigue of muscles called myasthenia. From the Greek word translated as weakness. In myasthenia muscles are weak, fatigue sets in at the slightest stress. The cause of the disease is not well understood, but it is believed that myasthenia gravis is a violation of the thymus gland, in which the blood receives a special type of autoimmune calf, changing the movement of nerve impulses to muscles. The disease most often affects the fairer sex. On average, the planet is sick 4 people from 100 thousand.

Mental fatigue. Asthenia

Mental fatigue is a very common complaint. In most cases, this condition is harmless and eliminated by taking adaptogens. But if the patient feels tired after resting, he suddenly increased temperature, pain and insomnia, decreases efficiency, more often diagnosed with fatigue. Asthenia can be observed both in physical and in mental illnesses.

From the point of view of medicine asthenia - a mental disorder in which the patient feels increased mental fatigue, body weakness, and instability emotional background. Very often, there is dizziness, pain in the joints or muscles.

Asthenia may be a combination of very different symptoms, so there may be a dislike of bright lights, sounds, smells some. The patient becomes very sensitive to pain. Some patients become very sensitive and disturbing, others on the contrary lethargic and indifferent to everything. If the violation is not related to the disease of the body, it is meant functional asthenia, which develops after severe shocks, after pregnancy and childbirth, with the use of alcohol and drugs. Cause of fatigue can be set and the use of medicaments: they may be hormonal contraceptive pills, hypnotics, antihistamines, antipsychotics, tranquilizers, antihypertensive.

If asthenic features combined with an increase in body temperature, fever, sweating, increased cervical lymph nodes, and all of these ailments last from six months and longer, they may be the sole manifestation of encephalitis. Sometimes after myocardial enterovirus, mononucleosis, adenovirus, and other diseases could also be observed asthenic syndrome. Another cause of mental fatigue may be a violation of metabolic processes. To clarify the diagnosis in this case should be tested for glucose, creatinine and electrolytes.

Fatigue Eye. Asthenia

Usually the cause of asthenia is prolonged or constant voltage bodies near vision, i.e. reading, writing something. Also there is the possibility of eyestrain when properly matched lenses glasses.

Symptoms:

- Pain in the eyes,
- Headache,
- The complexity of focus vision.

If the above symptoms appear suddenly, they can indicate the presence of glaucoma. Therefore, you should visit an ophthalmologist consultation.

After a while the vision in asthenia falls, the patient begins to squint hard to distinguish distant objects, it would be hard to read.

In order to facilitate the work of the organs of vision, it is necessary to do exercises for the eyes. For example, every hour on the computer do rest for a few minutes and look into the distance (in the box). Take comprehensive vitamin and mineral preparations, including vitamins E, A, B2 and B6, amino acids taurine and L-cysteine, minerals selenium, copper, zinc and chromium.

But the main thing when eyestrain - it's not to overload the eye. Before going to bed to do a compress with cold water or ice on the eye area, keeping it 10 - 15 minutes. You can make a poultice and day.

Spring Fatigue

In the spring, many people of all ages suffer from depression and fatigue. Reduced emotional background - perfect breeding ground for various diseases, including nerve.

The reason for the spring blues may be the lack of UV, oxygen, lack of exercise. Four times increases the probability of occurrence of this syndrome in those who spent the winter, "lying on the stove." Such people easily get sick, they have reduced capacity for work, get tired more quickly, pulling them to sleep.

Assist the body the vitamins found in foods: liver, meat, milk, fruits and vegetables, lean fat. This vitamins C, D, A, B complex, folic acid, beta-carotene. They activate the work of many systems, tone. Physical activity - it is also a wonderful remedy for loss of strength of the spring. Walking in the fresh air, contrasting water treatments to help regulate the nervous system improve the condition of blood vessels and strengthen the immune system.

In order to reassure shaky nerves can take peony tincture, motherwort, valerian. This will strengthen the body in dealing with stress; will not give way to despondency and despair. And at the same time and avoid the aggravation of various diseases of the digestive tract, which is usually seen on the background of shattered nervous system.

During Pregnancy

Fatigue - this is a very common complaint of pregnant women, which is often observed after the appearance of a baby into the world. If under normal lifestyle, good nutrition and taking drugs to relieve the state of fatigue persists, it may be a pathological condition. Such phenomena are not uncommon in the first and third trimesters. Woman have to say about the complaints the doctor and undergo a thorough examination.

The deterioration of the general state of health in the first trimester of pregnancy and often leads to the appearance of fatigue, bad mood, which usually take place after a good rest. If the feeling of fatigue does not pass, it should be examined by a doctor. If it is combined with a decrease in body weight, dysfunction of any of the bodies, the woman should be referred to hospital. Suffice pronounced fatigue in multiple pregnancies, in which case it is often seen in the background of high blood pressure, polycystic ovaries or violation of hormonal status. Sluggish and powerless, and those future moms who have strong toxicosis, there is a frequent and severe vomiting in the first trimester.

In the second and third trimesters of a woman's body weight is significantly increased, which also affects the general condition and the cause of fatigue. Very often there are violations of the digestive system, pain in the muscles and bones, itching, sleep disturbance. These abnormalities usually disappear on their own after a good rest. Very quickly tired women with impaired renal function, polyhydramnios, fatty liver, infectious jaundice. Worse tolerate these conditions nulliparous women.

What if the woman quickly gets tired exhausted, but she has no physiological abnormalities?

1. Sleep 8 - 9 hours a day, the best time to travel from 22 to 7 in the morning.

2. Before going to bed is useful to take a walk, go to the pool or make light exercises.

3. Before going to sleep well ventilate the room.

4. Take a shower before going to bed.

5. Drink 200 ml slightly warmed milk with a spoon of honey.

6. Eat a piece of cooked turkey - tryptophan is present in it a substance that improves sleep.

7. Sleep convenience to use several small pillows. Put them between your knees, under your lower back or as a convenience.

8. Rest for half an hour after lunch.

9. Eat a balanced way, to monitor the availability of vitamins in the diet. Very useful spinach, apples, apricots, currants, rose hips, pomegranates, buckwheat, rye bread, carrot.

The Child Has

Fatigue is not explainable by external causes; usually it says that the baby will become sick. Sometimes a child and weak after illness, but usually children activity normalized quickly. The longest the child's body recovered after some viruses, such as remitting fever. The first signs of the disease is a pain in the throat. Lethargy and weakness after such a disease may last several months.

If a child gets tired quickly, often drinks and urinates profusely, it may indicate the presence of diabetes. With the combination of the above symptoms with a decrease in body weight and epigastric, pain should visit a doctor immediately. If the child is recovering from a viral infection and is experiencing weakness, no special measures to strengthen it does not need. The body normalizes its work itself after some time. Just be spared child more, its activity should be feasible.

Often the cause of fatigue is the emotional overload. When such problems a child may disorder the work of many systems. The kid can sleep badly, be hyperactive, and refuse to visit a childcare institution. Maybe the cause of fatigue and lack of sleep. If fatigue is observed in adolescents, but this may not have anything to worry about. This is quite natural: the activity of phase changes to passive phase. There are a number of medicines that can suppress the child's energy.

At the use of any medications should talk with your doctor about possible side effects. One of the common causes of fatigue is anemia children. A blood test will give an accurate answer to the question of its presence. Chronic infections also significantly reduce the vigor of the child.

Diagnostics

In that case, if the fatigue is combined with nosebleeds, fainting, migraine states, vertigo, the patient is required to pass inspection.

The following methods are used for both adults and children can be assigned:

- Electroencephalogram,
- MRI
- Daily study of blood pressure,
- Inspection of a condition of the fundus,
- Scanning the neck vessels and transcranial duplex head,
- Interview with a psychologist,
- Tests for hormone levels, blood chemistry, urinalysis and blood immunogram,
- Sometimes you need a cardiologist, a gastroenterologist, and other professionals.

THREE STAGES OF ADRENAL FATIGUE

Few people know that is the adrenal glands. An average healthy person absolutely no reason to think about the different organs - they just have a good run and everything.

It's like a car - as he goes, you can't think, from what parts he is. Just sit behind the wheel, to refuel the car and going.

But when starting any health problems, then here it is necessary to study the structure of their "car" - his own body.

So, on the adrenal little known. And what is the hormones of the adrenal glands - is generally a dark forest! What are they, how many, for what they are - it's just a higher mathematics, a normal person inaccessible!

I raise this topic in view of the fact that the adrenal glands of women suffer while taking hormonal contraceptives. To understand the operation of these glands often-just need to, because they are responsible for adapting to stress, take care of all the blows of life and know their status is vital.

In clinical practice often encountered diseases caused by stress. Adrenal glands act as stress glands of the body - a reserve to be used when the body is under stress. Your energy, resistance, endurance depend on their proper functioning. Weakness of the adrenal glands can occur when the stress exceeds the body's ability to compensate for the stress and recover from it.

There are four main categories of stress:

Physical stress - hard work or too high physical exertion, lack of sleep, etc.

Chemical stress - from environment pollution, a diet rich refined carbohydrates, allergies to foods or additives, the imbalance of the endocrine glands.
Heat stress - overheating or overcooling of the body.
Emotional or mental stress.

In early studies, Hans Seelie defined patterns of diseases caused by stress. He opened the sequence of events, which are a response to chronic stress. This sequence of events known as the General Adaptation Syndrome CCA (General Adaptation Syndrome).

He identified three stages:

1. **Stage anxiety**. The initial chain of physical and chemical reactions caused by the interaction of the brain, nervous system and hormones, causing a surge of adrenal activity. They begin to work harder in response to a stressful situation has arisen, in fact this state adrenal exhaustion. After the initial alarm reaction, your body needs a recovery phase, which lasts 24-48 hours. At this time made less cortisol, the body has a lower ability to response to stress. At this stage, you feel fatigue, lethargy, and a desire to relax. If the stress continues for a long time, the adrenal glands will eventually be depleted. Sometimes in such cases, the patient goes to the doctor with symptoms adrenal exhaustion.

2. **Stage of resistance (resistance)**. After some time, the adrenal glands of the ongoing stress begin to adapt and restructure. They have a good ability to grow in size and functional activity. Prolonged anxiety reaction begins as adrenal exhaustion leading to adrenal exhaustion, which then goes back into a state of resistance to adrenal exhaustion stage. This resistance stage may last for months or even 15-20 years. Adrenal hormone cortisol is responsible for this stage. It stimulates the conversion of proteins, fats and carbohydrates into energy via gluconeogenesis, providing energy after glucose reserves depleted in the liver and muscles. Cortisol also provides the desired sodium level

needed to maintain blood pressure and heart function. If the stress continues for a long time or is very intense, resistance stage can go to the third stage.

3. **Stage of exhaustion**. This is the stage when a person loses the ability to adapt to stress. Adrenal function at this point sharply limited, and may set total disruption of bodily functions. The two main causes of the depletion of sodium ions are lost (due to lower aldosterone) and reduction of glucocorticoid hormones, like cortisol, leading to a decrease in gluconeogenesis, rapid hypoglycemia, loss of sodium and potassium retention. At the same time, insulin level is still high. Weakness appears. With a lack of energy, a reaction requiring energy, slow down. This is the stage when a person is likely to see a doctor, because the symptoms are no longer held.

Stress often comes as a result of events such as the death of loved ones, serious illness or accident. But he may also not so obvious way, as a result of tooth root infection, influenza, increased physical activity, quarrels with relatives, environment toxins, poor diet and other factors. If such events occur at the same time, accumulate or become chronic, and adrenal there is no possibility for a full recovery, adrenal weakness may occur as a result.

The hormones produced by the adrenal glands, have an impact on all the major physiological processes in our body: utilization of carbohydrates and fats, the conversion of fats and proteins into energy, the distribution of reserves of fat, regulating blood sugar, and the digestive tract and the cardiovascular system, the protective activity of anti-inflammatory and antioxidant hormones, allocated by the adrenal glands in order to minimize the adverse and allergic reactions to alcohol, drugs, food and environment toxins.

Weakness of the adrenal gland, or adrenal exhaustion became widespread, but rarely diagnosed disorder in the last 50 years. Despite the fact that it has been described in medical textbooks still 1800, and despite the development of effective treatment in the 1930s, most conventional doctors do not even know that such a problem exists.

Stress

Adrenal role is to protect the body from stress. Too many "small" stress leads to their exhaustion.

The main reason for the stress that overwhelms adrenal BOWL STAMINA:

- *Chronic lack of sleep.*
- *Violation of daily / light sleep-wake rhythms: shift work or going to bed late at night.*
- *Over-emotional and physical activity: hard work, divorce, financial problems, care for an elderly person or a child, intense physical training.*
- *Prolonged or severe disease. It's hard to say what comes first: the severity of the disease due to adrenal weakness or damage due to severe illness.*
- *Acute and chronic infection or pain.*
- *Surgical intervention.*
- *Root canal treatment.*
- *Injury.*
- *Depression. Again, I do not know what comes first.*
- *The reaction to life situations in the form of feelings of rage, fear, anxiety and guilt.*
- *Exposure to extreme temperatures (the ancient Chinese knew about it).*
- *Constant contact with toxins (household and environmental toxins).*
- *Deficiency of vitamins and other nutrients in the diet.*
- *Wrong selection of products: hobby products made with white flour, sugar and other refined products, as well as the scant amount of vegetables in the diet.*
- *The constant pursuit of excellence and overcome its capacity.*
- *The lack of pleasant events in life, such as meeting with friends, travel, etc..*

- *Allergy and / or intolerance to food or chemical agents. Products provocateurs lead to chronic intestinal inflammation. The adrenal glands respond to the "wrong" product of the reaction of stress in the form of increased levels of insulin and cortisone.*
- *Abuse of caffeine and sugary foods.*

Even if the diet is poor in carbohydrates and calories, it is unnecessary weight gain if you eat food, which is sensitive to the body. The sensitivity / intolerance of a product is not always easy to determine. As a result, chronic inflammation of the body is formed, which keeps the adrenal glands on edge.

From school it's known that the adrenal glands react to danger / stress reaction of "fight or flight". Now of danger to life increases the frequency of heart rate and blood pressure to increase blood flow to the heart, muscles and brain.

At the same time blocks the digestion, the immune system, as well as other organs and systems that are not needed for emergency rescue.

Unfortunately, humanity today is in a "fight or flight" mode too often. It is much longer than was intended by Mother Nature.

Our ancestors did not meet every day with saber-toothed tiger. If a person did not treat a predator, then adrenal recovery he had enough time. Man of the civilized world has to, figuratively speaking, "fight and flight" dozens and sometimes hundreds of times a day.

Now tell me, who is now the adrenal glands are in good shape?

Adrenal exhaustion, as the main organ of survival, pulled by an immune system, endocrine glands, and other organs and systems. Here are a few examples where nobody would never think of the adrenal glands.

Stress hormone cortisone is able to destructive actions with respect to the proteins of the human body. The result is a loss of muscle mass and / or bone density (osteoporosis). Cortisone steals proteins in bone and muscle tissue to use as fuel: sugar.

If the "product" of the body's proteins, sugar not used for energy needs, it will not return back, and settles in the fat tissue around the waist. The "melting" a result of constant theft of proteins from muscle tissue as a result of constant stress, muscle arms, legs and buttocks. But it is impossible to fasten the trousers at the waist.

High cortisone may explain why some people can not lose weight on high-protein diet.

This is because the hormone cortisone stress gracefully blocks the action of hormones, fat burners. In constant survival mode body "thinks" that it is better to save up energy reserves around the waist.

And here's another sobering fact: during stress, in anticipation of a real or imaginary fights (the adrenal glands do not distinguish the former from the latter), there is a spasm of vessels in the skin. Since adrenal glands are prepared to defend the body against possible bleeding from his injuries.

It is easy to imagine what will be the quality of the skin of those who are exposed to multiple stresses.

ONE OF ALARMS HEAVY adrenal exhaustion is a sudden penetrating pain in the lower back.

In my view, it is wiser not to wait for the "stab in the back" by the adrenal glands and now once again to revise the above-mentioned causes of stress and outline an action plan to facilitate the share of the adrenal glands. I, on the other hand, will help reader's inaccessible knowledge.

Fatigue

This syndrome is very easily confused with other conditions and diseases. Moreover, there is no specific test for diagnosis.

Below I gave the symptoms, which usually appear in people with tired adrenal glands. Symptoms of this syndrome is very easily confused with symptoms of hypothyroidism.

- You can no longer tolerate stressful situations easily, as they are transferred earlier. Try to avoid conflicts and emotional situations.
- You can be difficult to concentrate.
- You annoy elementary stuff.
- You have a weak immune system, and you often get sick.
- Do you have a stomach ulcer and / or 12-duodenum?
- You constantly feel tired, because no matter how long you slept. You wake up tired already.
- You have low blood pressure without apparent reason.
- You often cold.
- You are suffering frequent headaches and migraines.
- Do you suffer from allergies?
- You can't lose weight no matter how you try.
- Do you have a craving for salty, sweet foods and caffeine?

As I always like to say "with hormones to be trifled with, and usually no good, they do not stop." And when the glands themselves are not functioning properly, and from there, like a snowball begins to accumulate one problem after another.

Hormonal Imbalance

When the adrenal glands are tired, they are no longer able to control the stress hormone - cortisol in the blood, and remains a high level. This prevents the excretion of excess estrogen from our body. Estrogen in turn, increases the amount of special-thyroid binding globulin, which are attached to the hormones secreted by the thyroid gland. When thyroid hormones globulin attached to it, they are in an inactive form, whereby our body can't use them in the blood and their level is significantly reduced. Just for this reason, symptomatic RLS is very similar to hypothyroidism.

Weak immunity

Tired adrenal glands weaken the immune system and its proper functioning. There is a weakening of protective mechanisms, such as for example in our intestines. The barrier, which prevents the ingress of food particles through the intestinal wall into the blood stream weakens and develops one of the main causes of allergies and autoimmune diseases - syndrome of increased intestinal permeability.

Violation of the hypothalamic-pituitary-adrenal coordination

This special reaction network controls our reaction to stress and trauma, temperature control, digestion, mood, libido and energy.

Exhaustion

What causes adrenal exhaustion?

Depletion of the adrenal glands exist as long as humanity exists, but it has reached epidemic proportions only in the last 100 years around the world, and about 30 years in the post. Why is this happening? The answer lies in our lifestyle, which, over time, has changed. The level of the average man stress, nutrition and toxic load is higher and higher, when compared to the same data with the beginning of the twentieth century.

At the simplest level, adrenal depletion caused by the failure of the adrenal glands, to cope with stress. But in order to truly understand our condition, we need to know how your adrenal glands reached that point. We instinctively feel that our adrenal glands are not working optimally, but what is the reason for this?

On this page, I am going to list the main cause's adrenal exhaustion. This is by no means an exhaustive list, but I think it covers approximately 90% suffering from adrenal exhaustion. Some of you can identify two or three of the list of reasons that relate to you, but, in reality, adrenal exhaustion may be caused by a single factor.

You should also understand that adrenal exhaustion does not occur abruptly. For this purpose, as a rule, it takes years until your adrenals are exhausted. So when you're looking for the cause of the symptoms of adrenal exhaustion, take a look at a few years in your past. Physical or emotional trauma, which occurred five - ten years ago, may be the most factor that started the downward spiral of exhaustion.

REASON # 1: Emotional stress

The number one reason for exhaustion of the adrenal glands, without a doubt, stress. And, as you know, stress can come from any area of your life. Whether it's personal life, which is falling apart, unjust boss, moving to a new city or sleepless nights spent at the head of a newborn baby with colic, the effect is the same. It is a kind of low-intensity stress, which is not particularly affected in the short term, but can have dire consequences for our health in the long term.

There are many strategies to cope with stress, but it is best to simply remove the cause. This often means the beginning of a new relationship or a career change to a more pleasant. Sometimes, all you need to do, just apply some organizational tools to simplify your life. Take a step back and think about what makes you truly happy.

REASON # 2: DIET

We consume more sugar than ever consumed. In fact, over the past 200 years, the consumption of sugar has increased from 500-600 grams per year, up almost 72 kilograms. Our genetics during this period has not changed since our body to cope with all those extra calories. Answer: We produce more cortisol and insulin, which increases the load on the pancreas and adrenal glands.

There is another connection between sugar and adrenal exhaustion. I eat too much sugar, and just rack the weight, we know very well. But did you know that being overweight can also be a factor contributing to adrenal exhaustion? Just think what additional load created extra 25 - 50 kg of your body and internal organs? If being overweight makes you feel tired, there is a chance that it just makes your tired adrenal glands.

REASON # 3: Lack of sleep

If you are trying to find a balance between work and personal life and realize that you just can't fit into a day, you're probably not getting enough sleep. Our ancestors could afford to nine hours of sleep a day healthy, but these days, some of us may not be counted, and half of that. The average American sleeps 6.1

hours a day, but those who are in the early stages of adrenal exhaustion, often sleep less.

Why is it important? The long, peaceful sleep is exactly what your body needs to repair itself. The body has a fantastic ability to repair itself, but it is a miracle takes time. Keep at least 7-8 hours of sleep (or sleep longer, if you need to), and the likelihood that you will suffer adrenal exhaustion will be much less

REASON # 4: CHEMICALS AND POLLUTION

I mentioned "the burden toxins" in the first paragraph of this article. When I say this, I mean the overall level of toxicity that we face in everyday life. The toxins in our food, pollutants in the air, the chlorine in our drinking water, antibiotics in our meat and pesticides in our vegetables ... It increases our load of toxins.

Each year, about 2,000 different chemicals introduced to the consumer market. Some of them get into our food in the products that we buy, but very few of them are fully tested to ensure the safety of people. However, these chemicals and toxins, ultimately, can lead to serious diseases such as Alzheimer's disease, cancer, or heart disease. But even if you do not suffer from these diseases, they may have a significant impact on the quality of your life, your immune system, digestion and more.

How does this affect your adrenal glands? It is known that many of these chemicals directly violate adrenal function. Often your body (in particular, other parts of the HPA axis) adapted to compensate. But if you continue to overstrain your adrenal glands over a long period, adrenal exhaustion becomes the most likely outcome.

REASON # 5: Chronic Disease

When we talk about long-term stress, our adrenal glands, we must not forget to include in the list of chronic diseases. If you suffer from asthma, arthritis, and diabetes, they impose on your adrenal glands requirements, which are much higher than normal. When you are suffering from these diseases for a long period, your adrenal glands become overworked and tired. You should also know that the treatment of chronic diseases, too, is often too stressful for the body.

Other diseases that can weaken the adrenal glands is fibromyalgia, Lyme disease, various parasites and any condition causing chronic pain.

REASON # 6: TRAUMA

Depletion of the adrenal glands can be caused not only by long-term factors - severe physical trauma can also cause adrenal exhaustion. It used to be that the only physically traumatic incident may not have any long-term effects beyond the obvious scars and wounds. But now we obtained proof that the injuries have a much more lasting impact on our health and can affect such things as hormonal balance and the adrenal glands, many years later.

I'm not just talking about an accident or other incident. Large operations also fall under this category as this extraordinary stress on the body. If you can trace the connection of their individual symptoms with the traumatic event in the past, it is quite possible that you have found the root cause of your adrenal exhaustion.

RECOVERY TREATMENT

Diagnosis and treatment

Current diagnosis of adrenal diseases include a variety of methods. The main are the following common diagnostic techniques:

- Laboratory blood samples for analysis of hormone levels
- Ultrasound adrenal gland
- Magnetic resonance imaging
- CT scan
- Laboratory tests of blood and urine.

It's also used by numerous research methods with the contrast to identify or rule out the presence of the tumor. As the most informative method can be noted MSCT adrenal or also well-established method of diagnosis - MRI of the adrenal glands.

By definition, aldosterone levels, free cortisol and other hormones in the daily urine can set various diseases of the kidneys and adrenal glands, as different degeneration, hormone-dependent tumors, and inflammatory diseases more. It is important to take steps to make it work at full strength gland.

At a high level of in formativeness are diagnostic methods, which include the latest developments in cancer radiotherapy semiotics directly dependent on their hormonal activity. In this regard, it is considered to be very effective methods of radiation research cortex and brain structures of the adrenal glands and surrounding tissue. An example of radiation diagnosis can serve scintigraphy.

Speaking about the treatment of adrenal diseases, not to mention the following modern and proven methods and techniques to effectively treat the adrenal glands. Imagine an exemplary sequence of actions if the adrenal glands are sore.

For example, the main method of visualization is Addison's disease adrenal computed tomography in the abdominal cavity and to determine the condition of the affected organ. This study also helps differentiate other pathological conditions, for example, if the liver colitis. According to established practice, when there is a malfunction of an internal organ, carried out for the diagnosis of CT, MRI or any other instrumental examination of patients.

An important place in the study of the kidneys and their appendages takes preparation for MRI or ultrasound to and other forms of examination. Good to know that before the ultrasound requires bowel cleansing to accumulate fecal do not create obstacles to the visualization.

If you suspect a malignant tumor, prepare laboratory histological preparation. To do this laparoscopically fence made of a tissue sample of the affected organ, and study its histology for the detection of cancer cells.

Modern endocrinology offers patients comprehensive assistance when a problem is detected with the adrenal glands. When the sick goes to a medical facility, doctor suggests the initial phase of its survey, and only after a detailed review of inspection results prescribe treatment.

If the patient is found to adrenal damage, then the appointed conservative treatment of a variety of drugs. Hormone replacement therapy is indicated only in the worst cases, when you can't cure hormonal preparations, removes the adrenal gland.

But not everything comes to an end only in the operating room. Existing methods of pharmacotherapy and the newest drugs can achieve significant results. Violation of the adrenal gland in the initial stage of the process is successfully corrected by the introduction of hormones in the form of drugs. Adrenal folk remedies Treatment also can achieve significant improvement in the patient's condition. In this method of treatment effects on the organism almost not expressed.

NATURAL WAYS TO TREAT ADRENAL FATIGUE

Treatment of adrenal folk remedies quite popular, because here you will need a minimum cost, and all the ingredients can be found even at home. The adrenal glands are part of the endocrine system and the hormones involved in the production of different purposes. If such a development would be disrupted, the body starts to seriously suffer, and then without the aid no longer do.

If the diagnosis is not as such, but there is a feeling that the adrenal glands begin to not work properly, it is worth trying a few recipes from the national stockpile, which will help normalize all the functions:

1. Boil the honey garlic, pound, and there is 1 tbsp. gruel with complete impotence or fatigue.

2. Take 100 grams. herb astragals (not dried), add 1 liter. red table wine, to keep for 21 days in the closet, shaking from time to time. To pass through a sieve and drink 30 oz. morning, afternoon and evening for 30 minutes before a meal.

3. Take an empty bottle, put it as chopped beets, as will fit without ramming, pour vodka. Keep 2 weeks in the pantry. Drink 25 ml once per day on an empty stomach. This tool will help relieve fatigue and restore activity.

4. 200 grams. bran in 1 liter fill. boiling water, boil for 60 minutes, decant through cheesecloth. Drink 3 - 4 times a day on an empty stomach.

5. Finely chopped celery, add 200 ml of water at room temperature, to sustain 2 h. Split into several doses per day and drink. Very good tones.

6. Every day to drink 100 ml of freshly squeezed beet juice 3 times a day.

7. Fresh leaves cranberries used instead of tea leaves.

8. Drink a strong green tea. Replace them any other drinks.

9. Black tea with milk and honey.

10. Drink infusion of peppermint tea instead.

11. Drink pomegranate juice.

12. Drink grape juice in 100 ml, divide it into small portions: a sip every 120 minutes.

13. Eat cabbage cleft to activate the body.

14. Eat sacred lotus. Are eaten all parts of the plant.

15. Underground parts and flowers Saranac activates and improves appetite. The plant can be dry, grind into flour and make cakes of it.

16. 2 tsp Icelandic moss pour 400 ml of water at room temperature, put on fire and let boil. Immediately remove, let cool, pass through a sieve. Drink the resulting number over 24 hours. You can make the broth: 25 g. raw materials 750 ml of boiling water. Cook for half an hour, passed through a sieve and drink per day.

17. Grind 1 lemon with rind, mixed with a few slices of grated garlic, put in a 0.5 liter. bottle. Add water at room temperature up to the top. Under the hood, hold for four

days in a closet. Then rearrange the cold. Drink 1 tablespoon in the morning 20 minutes before a meal.

18. Take 24 lemons, 0.4 kg of garlic. Crush garlic, from lemons to make juice, all combined and put into a glass bottle. Cover with a cloth. Drink once a day for a teaspoon of warm water.

19. 1 tbsp. Astragals fluffy flowering pour 200 ml of boiling water, hold for 3 hours to eat 2 tablespoons 4 - 5 times a day 60 minutes before meals.

20. 2 tbsp. Knotweed pour 1 liter. of boiling water and keep 120 minutes. Through a sieve, honey and put to use, 200 ml three times a day on an empty stomach.

21. 3 tbsp. black currant leaves pour two cups of boiling water for two hours. Drink 100 ml three - five times a day before meals.

22. Make an infusion of red clover flowers. Drink tea instead of with impotence.

23. Two tablespoons of chopped root of wild carrots pour 500 ml of boiling water. After 2 hours passed through a sieve and consume 100 ml three times a day.

24. Take 3 tbsp. chopped straw oats; pour 400 ml of boiling water. Hold to cool. Drink per day.

25. 2 teaspoons juniper cones pour 400 ml of water at room temperature; hold 2 hours to pass through a sieve. Drink 1 tablespoon 3 - 4 times a day.

26. 2 tbsp. chickweed herb brew 500 ml of boiling water, hold 60 minutes. Passed through a sieve and drink 50 - 70 ml three times a day 60 minutes before meal.

27. 1 tbsp. nasturtium (green parts) to brew 200 ml of boiling water, hold 60 - 120 minutes, drink 2 tablespoons three times a day on an empty stomach.

28. 3 tsp calliopsis grass pour 400 ml boiling water, leave for 60 - 120 minutes, pass through a sieve and drink 100 ml of warm to three times a day on an empty stomach.

29. Dry the underground parts of snowdon rose, grind and add the alcohol (70%) in the proportions: 10 gr. raw materials of 100 ml of alcohol. Drink 15 - 20 drops three times a day.

30. 50 grams. dry Hypercom pour 500 ml of Cahors wine, put on half an hour on a steam bath. Drink a tablespoon three times a day before meals for a week - one and a half.

31. Boil the potatoes in their skins, you can slightly not boil. Eat in the cold broth, 200 ml every two days.

32. 20 grams. chicory root pour a glass of boiling water. Boil for 10 minutes, pass through a sieve and use one tablespoon every 4 hours. You can pour 20 g. 0.1 l fresh roots. alcohol. Hold 10 days in the pantry. Drink 20 drops five times a day.

33. 20 gr. Chinese magnolia fruit, pour a glass of boiling water. Drink a tablespoon three times a day slightly warmed. Before eating or four hours after a meal.

Vitamins

Due to the fact that the cause of fatigue is often a shortage of vitamins, an excellent preparation for the normalization of the brewer's yeast are. Today they are available in a convenient form of tablets or capsules. Yeast contain vitamins B1, B6, B2, B9, PP, H, vitamin E. In addition, in yeast contains essential amino acids and fatty acids (linoleic acid, oleic acid and arachidonic) and trace elements: manganese, zinc, iron, magnesium, calcium.

Brewer's yeast, due to the large number of biologically active substances that have a beneficial effect on the body:

- Improve digestion,
- Improve immunity,
- Strengthen the body, located in the extreme conditions,
- Help to clean the fabric of the products of metabolism,
- Prevent allergic phenomenon, osteoporosis, tooth decay,
- Regulate the nervous system.

The drug is indicated for adult patients, it does not cause any discomfort. The only contraindication is idiosyncrasy to beer yeast. Taking the drug for a month, and then make a break for 15 days and can be just one course of treatment.

Water treatment procedures

1. Take a bath with a water temperature of 37.5 degrees. You can simply hold it in warm water feet.

2. The bucket pour water temperature 45 - 50 degrees, more - water at room temperature. First 5 minutes to lower legs in the first bucket, then a minute into the second. To do so five times. Then make a foot massage with cream or camphor alcohol.

3. Every day, pour or sponge oneself down with cold water. Most useful to do this procedure in the morning.

4. If intellectual work is helpful to do before going to bed a hot bath (water temperature 42 degrees) for the legs. This will help pull blood from the brain to the legs.

5. Take a bath with pine extract. To make homemade extract should collect twigs, cones and needles of conifers, add room

temperature water and boil on low heat for half an hour. Then remove from heat, cover and leave overnight. If the extract is made according to the rules, it must be dark chocolate color. On acceptance of a bath rather 0,75. extract.

6. Mix 20 gr. black currant leaves, 60 g. raspberry leaf, 10 grams. thyme, 10 g. Woodruff shoots. Mix well and brew boiling water. Hold 15 minutes, after which the bath can be used.

Honey Treatment

1. Eat every day honey with pollen (pollen).

2. Stir in 200 ml of water, 2 tsp honey, add 2 tsp poppy petals and boil for 5 minutes. Drink a teaspoon in the morning, afternoon and evening.

3. Combine 250 ml May honey, 150 ml of aloe juice and 350 ml of Cahors. Flower of aloe vera before collecting leaves do not water for three days. After mixing, the ingredients should be kept in the refrigerator for 7 days. Drink one tablespoon in the morning, afternoon and evening for half an hour before a meal with impotence.

4. Before breakfast, drink 1 tsp Lemon juice mixed with 1 tsp honey and 1 tbsp. vegetable oil.

5. Mix 1300 gr. honey, 150 gr. kidney birch, 200 ml of olive oil, 50 g. linden flowers, 1 tbsp. finely chopped leaves of aloe. The warm honey aloe. Buds of birch and linden flowers to brew a small amount of water on the fire to warm up for 2 minutes, mixed with honey, stir in butter. Keep cold. Drink 2 tablespoons morning, afternoon and evening, mixing prior to use.

6. Combine 1 tsp dried calamus root milled with the same amount of honey. Eat after breakfast and after dinner.

7. Mix 0.5 kg of walnuts, 100 grams. aloe juice, juice of 3 lemons, 0.3 kg of honey. Eat 1 tsp three times a day for half an hour before a meal.

8. Liter jar pour 0.1 kg of honey, 150 g. finely chopped onion, pour wine to the brim. Leave in a closet for 15 days. To pass through a sieve and drink every day for 3 tbsp.

CHOOSE PROPER DIET

The adrenal glands are small glands located above the kidneys, than, in fact, due to their name. Despite the small size of these glands, they perform a very important function - to produce hormones, without which man can't live, including sex hormones, adrenaline, cortisol and aldosterone.

The problems can be eliminated by treatment of adrenal dysfunction. Along with the reduction of chronic stress, regulation of our emotional reactions to stressors, as well as a change in power can deal with adrenal fatigue.

Therefore, I propose to your attention the recommendations for food, which is not only a positive effect on the adrenal glands, but also increase energy levels and improve your sleep.

The right time for adrenal health food

If we spend a long time without food, our adrenal glands are hard at work, producing more cortisol and adrenaline in order to maintain the normal functioning of the body. If over time the blood sugar level is lowered, this causes the stress response. It is therefore important to know that our body needs energy, even during sleep. Cortisol plays an important role in the regulation of sugar levels in the body, so it is important to make healthy food and do it on time.

Cortisol levels vary according to the circadian rhythm of the human: he begins to rise about 6 pm; the highest point reaches at 8 pm, and during the day cortisol levels can rise and fall in accordance with the body's needs. In the night cortisol level decreases and the lowest level of this hormone occurs during sleep.

Therefore, to maintain hormonal balance necessary to:

- more food should be consumed early in the day;
- more light food in smaller quantities to be taken by the end of the day;
- exercise can also increase cortisol levels, so the treatment of adrenal fatigue is recommended moderate activity;
- more intense exercises recommended in the morning or late afternoon when cortisol levels are elevated.

Why I do not want to eat in the morning?

Old as the world saying that the breakfast - the main meal of the day, in fact, true. Nutritious breakfast that contains protein, absorbed for an hour after getting up, helps to balance the metabolism and keep cortisol levels are normal throughout the day. However, it is difficult to "push" in the breakfast, if you do not want to eat at all, even though we know that this is necessary.

That's why in the morning do not want to have:

Corticotrophin-releasing hormone (CRH) can suppress appetite, quickly getting into the blood in the morning.
Reduced liver function may be accompanied by adrenal fatigue, which may also be the reason for lack of appetite in the morning.

Supply time for cortisol regulation throughout the day:

- Try to eat breakfast within an hour of lifting or 8 o'clock in the morning to restore blood sugar levels, which after a night downgraded.
- At 9 am, organize a healthy snack.
- Try to snack during the time interval from 11 am till noon, in order to prevent a decrease in cortisol levels.

- Grab a snack healthy food from 14 to 15, to smooth the drop in cortisol levels, which occurs approximately 15 to 16 hours. By the way, a lot of people at this time feel unexplained fatigue and somnolence and therefore extend over a cup of coffee or a carbohydrate-rich foods, which is not recommended, because it adversely affects the hormonal balance.
- Try to have dinner somewhere between 17 and 18 hours, and better suited for a dinner bland food. At first it will seem complex and unfamiliar, but your body is super responsive with time will get used to this dinner, and even love them.
- An hour before bedtime, too, can eat something light, but in any case it is "easy" should not contain refined sugar. In this role perfectly suited cheeses and vegetables.

Meals and drinks for the health of the adrenal glands

When a person is lowered blood sugar levels, it pulls on sweet. Unfortunately, if a person is struggling with adrenal fatigue with the help of cookies, candy, cola and / or coffee, obtained from such foods and beverages the energy is not "long-playing". What you get as a result: a sharp jump in the level of sugar in the blood, accompanied by the same leap of insulin levels, which suppresses a lightning surge sugar. And it is also stressful for the body.

Stress and exhaustion in combination with hunger can disrupt our ability to make healthy decisions. If we are not aware of how much caffeine and refined carbohydrates enters into our body, we do not understand how it affects our hormones and their work, along with sleep patterns.

So what foods are good for the adrenal glands:

- fresh whole organic foods, appropriate season (i.e. strawberry - that's fine, if it is collected in the summer in the garden, rather than bought in a supermarket in the winter);
- Avoid preservatives, hormonal additives, artificial colors and chemicals;
- include in your diet lean protein products that reduce cravings for caffeine and refined sugar;
- Try to always have a supply of ready-made snacks, so you can satisfy your hunger if necessary.

As for drinks, all very simple: the maximum limit the use of alcohol, caffeine and energy.

The role of the salt in the adrenal health:

You will be surprised, but his craving for salt time adrenal fatigue is not necessary to suppress. When adrenal insufficiency craving for salty associated with reduced levels of the steroid hormone aldosterone. This hormone helps the body to maintain the mineral metabolism and ion balance and regulate blood pressure.

When cortisol levels rise, aldosterone level drops.

Like cortisol, aldosterone levels vary throughout the day and is also subject to the effects of stress. Continuing low aldosterone levels can adversely affect the water-salt balance, and sodium intake helps to restore the balance.

By the way, dizziness in the morning or after a bath may be indicative of reduced blood pressure, which is a side effect of adrenal insufficiency. Relieving symptoms will help quality salt (for example, seawater).

Other nutrients needed for the health of the adrenal glands

Vitamins, minerals and trace elements play an important role in maintaining and restoring adrenal health and to maintain the entire endocrine system. The most important of these are:

- vitamins C, E and B (particularly B6 and pantothenic acid) help to regulate the levels of stress hormones;
- magnesium delivers energy to the adrenal glands;
- calcium and minerals, including zinc, manganese, iodine and selenium, have a calming effect on the body.

Also, special herbs can be used in the treatment of adrenal fatigue - adaptogenes that increase the body's resistance to stress.

And remember that eating a meal, but a doctor will still need to address. Constant fatigue can be a symptom of many diseases, not just adrenal fatigue. It is therefore necessary to pay due attention to other bodies in addition to taking care of the adrenal glands.

EPILOGUE

Supplement of my friend Kate

I suffered from tired adrenal syndrome, when passed through a very difficult period of stress in their lives, which eventually changed my life for the better. But I'm for it, you might say, have paid with their adrenal glands.

Restoration of normal function of these glands is necessary to begin slowly, do not change all at once in a single day, not irritate your body even more.

It has been a year since I have ceased to be nervous over nothing and finally I can normally sleep quality, and most importantly. I do not feel constantly tired and my mood is quite stable.

That's what I did in order to give my poor adrenal glands breathe freely:

- I stopped paying attention to stimuli that previously caused my negative emotions. Just I thought to myself, as if it will be so important in 5 years and usually the answer was clearly "no."

- I began practicing yoga, and special breathing pranayama. Once I started taking special Emotional Freedom Techniques, which I found with my doctor. Believe me, this is a very easy and effective practice of which, I believe, everyone should know.

- I stopped eating foods that are loaded adrenal glands. This sugar, simple carbohydrates, refined products and vegetable oils.

- I began to eat every 3 hours, in order to stabilize blood sugar levels and balance cortisol levels. Breakfast should be no later than 30 minutes after you wake up. And before going to bed -Small snack consisting of fat, such as coconut spoon or butter. In no case, do not practice intermittent fasting with tired adrenal glands!

- I started to eat more healthy fat and protein. My diet accounted for almost 80% of the calories of these two main components.

- I no longer indulge in salt. Salt as much as I liked. Of course, using natural Himalayan pink salt, and not the white dining room. The fact is that during times of stress, our body takes a large amount of salt, which is why many people experience cravings for pickles during stressful situations.

- I stopped to drink 2 liters of fluid a day. I saw only when feeling thirsty. Yes, it is absolutely contrary to all the tenets of healthy eating, but behind it there is a science. Excessive consumption of water and dilute salt our electrolytes in the blood, metabolism slows down and thyroid function. The easiest, as you can tell, if you do not get completely drunk - is to look to the toilet on the color of urine, it should not be transparent, and slightly yellow.

- I'm serious was the "lean" to one of the most important vitamins for the adrenal glands - Vitamin C, but not in the form of synthetic, not digestible ascorbic acid.

- I began to eat a large quantity of giblets, due to their high content of nutrients, especially vitamin A comes to 3 times a week.

- I began to go to bed at the same time and sleep at least 8 hours a day. In complete darkness.

- In a month, I ceased to engage in cardio, so as not to irritate your adrenals even further. I began to walk more.

- He began to eat and drink more fermented foods (sauerkraut, beet kvass, homemade yogurt), for the normalization of friendly bacteria and extra Vitamin C.

- I start taking magnesium and magnesium oil, a mineral which strongly leached during stress.

- I It began to take herbs that have a positive effect on the adrenal glands: licorice root, gingko biloba, Ashwagandha, Tulsi and Radiola.

- Increase the intake of omega-3, in order to combat chronic inflammation.

- Well, the most important and simple - to try to look at all the positive aspects, enjoy life and smile more often.

Finally

It took me more than six months to bring my adrenals to normal. So, please, do not count on immediate results. Natural methods are much slower drugs, but they are aimed at the root of the problem and treat the very cause and not just the symptoms. They have no side effects and does not "kill" the other organs and systems.

Try to stick to this way of life at least a month and as always observe how responsive and feel your body. Do your symptoms have improved, it is better if you were sleeping and to tolerate stress, you could start to lose those stubborn and hateful kilograms.

As with other invisible conditions, Tired Adrenal Syndrome goes hand in hand with insulin resistance and leptin resistance. All these states can and should be corrected by a proper diet and a healthy lifestyle.

Tired Adrenal Syndrome - not a myth but a very real pathological condition, which occurs in almost everyone and prevents us from fully enjoy and celebrate life.

Take control in your hands and let your poor adrenal glands rest. They definitely deserve this.

And what do you think - you have **ADRENAL FATIGUE?**

AUTHOR PAGE

My name is Jack Oliver and me the goal is to make your life easier in the perception. All you need is knowledge that will help you get out of a stressful and depressing situation. I like to help people. I hope my work was not in vain.

P.S. You need to be patient, to go the way of healing with maximum efficiency.

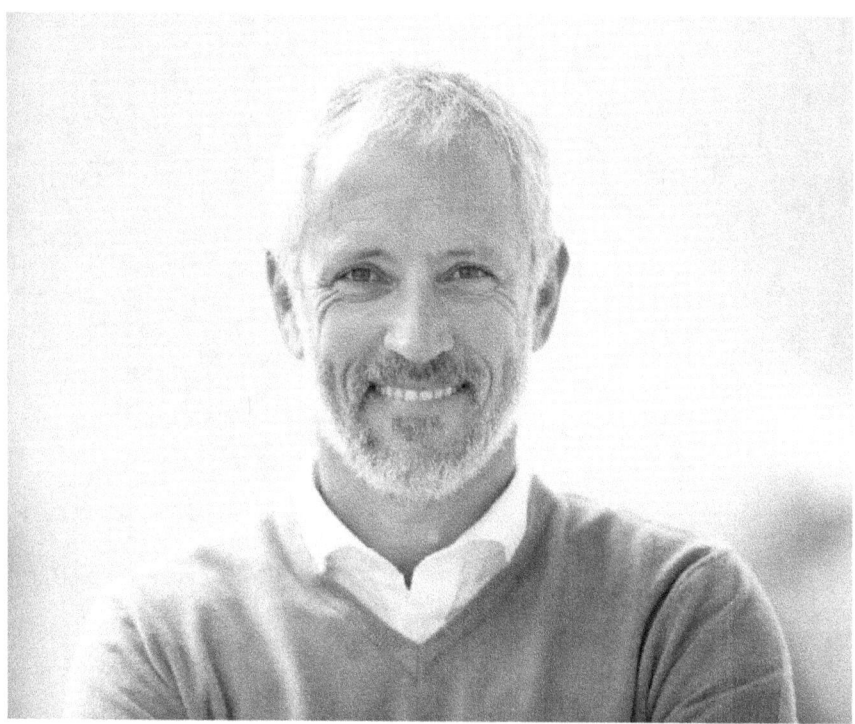

Please, leave a feedback about the book! This will help other customer to learn more about this content.

Thanks to you, Dear Reader and Good Luck!

CHECK OUT MY OTHER BOOKS, THAT ARE EXACTLY WILL HELP YOU:

Cognitive Behavioral Therapy

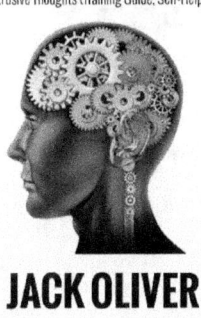

Unlimited Memory

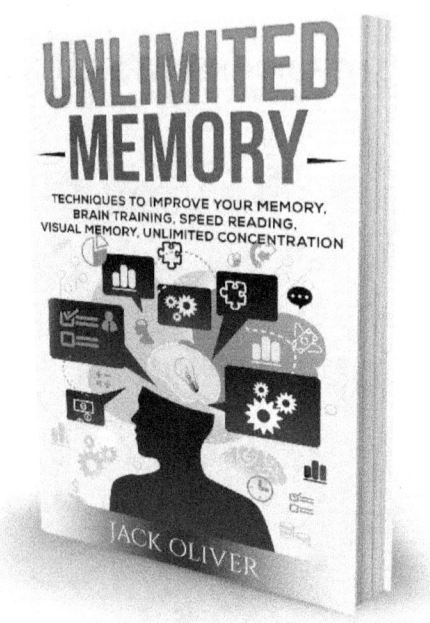

Social Confidence

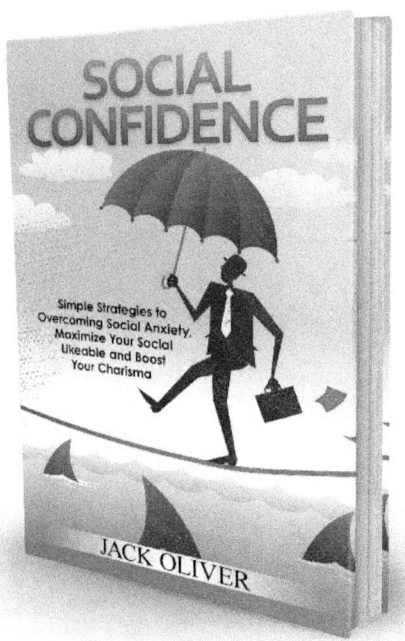

Be Strong!

www.ingramcontent.com/pod-product-compliance
Lightning Source LLC
Chambersburg PA
CBHW070402190526
45169CB00003B/1073